NIL BY MOUTH

By

Leslie John Curson

A day by day account of hospital routine and the intimate thoughts of a patient admitted for a prostatectomy.

CONTENTS

1. Tuesday May 4th

The day had at last arrived, 4th May 1982, for my admission into Sutton Hospital for the operation on my enlarged prostate gland.

My wife Joyce had agreed to accompany me and take my clothes away, leaving me with two pairs of pyjamas only and a dressing gown which were to be my main walk-about clothing for my estimated twelve days stay. Waiting outside "Traders Ward", which was the one to which I was allocated, I pondered on how it had been given its name. The answer lay in the inscribed wall plaque above my head, that it was indeed built by the Traders of Sutton at a cost of £5,000 and was dedicated to the men of Sutton who made the supreme sacrifice in the first world war 1914-1918.

The time now being 9.15am, and the doctors rounds completed, I sat waiting a bit apprehensively wondering what fate had in store, and whether the operation would be successful. A lady eventually approached asking if she could help us and upon learning I was to be admitted, led Joyce and I into the ward to a bed two down on the left. The screens were pulled around the bed and I was instructed to change into pyjamas and dressing gown, when I would be taken on a "tour" of the ward by the clerk, who I later knew was Eve.

Joyce, meanwhile, had collected my clothes together and put my personal bits and pieces and toiletries into the various cupboards, drawers and spaces on the bedside locker. With our 'goodbyes' completed and the promise to call in this evening during visiting time, Joyce left and I resigned myself to whatever lay ahead.

Eve, the ward clerk presented herself on cue and walked with me to the far end of the ward, through swing doors to the day room which housed a large TV set, and ample easy chairs. There were magazines, books, cards and dominoes for our enjoyment. Returning through the ward, the bathrooms and toilets were pointed out, not in too greater detail as that exploration would come later. Eve took my relevant papers and said that anything I wished to know, the staff would be only too willing to help, and at that left me to take stock of my surroundings.

The chap occupying the first bed space was sitting quietly observing me and it wasn't long before I was chatting with him and enquiring what he had been in for. I learnt his name was George and did not bother about surnames at this stage, as I noticed a small tab low down at the foot of the bed with his name.

A flat wooden box hanging at the end of the bed held my papers to record my temperature, blood pressure and pulse rate and another paper gave personal details and the tablets I was taking.

My first introduction to Charles, the ward orderly, was when he asked me to fill a bottle he handed me, with a urine sample. George had already briefed me not to call the ward orderly Charlie, which to me had its obvious reasons. I was in the act of attempting to put a reasonable amount in this bottle, when a nurse stuck her head through the screen opening, but quickly withdrew it. No doubt she'll be seeing more of me during the next week. Charles took my 'sample' which wasn't a lot, because I had recently been, and had some tests made on it, because when he came back, he said it was like maidens water, quite pure, which I assumed was a good sign. The medical registrar put in an appearance and asked the same questions he had asked on one of my previous visits to the hospital, so I hope he was satisfied by my answers this time.

George in the next bed had his prostate 'op' performed last Wednesday and was due to go out in a day or so. He had been there five weeks this Friday, because a blood disorder held up the operation until the doctors were satisfied it could go ahead. He told me he didn't remember coming round and in fact his wife had been to see him during the afternoon visiting and had been talking to him. Apparently when he finally recovered later that evening, he asked had his wife been in to see him and was quite amazed when told he had been talking to her.

In order to clear out my system before the operation, four Senokot tablets were given to me to wash down. I had only taken one of these several weeks previously prior to having an X-ray taken of my bladder regions, and was uncertain then as to how strong they were and had waited impatiently for something to happen. Nothing did, so it was hoped that when I was X-rayed it would not interfere with the process.

However, back to the present and four Senokots. I was left to wonder how rapidly they would work and whether I'd make the toilet in time.

About 10.20, the tea and coffee trolley moved slowly down the ward, and as I had instructions to drink plenty, I had one. The empty beds were slowly filling up with new arrivals, so it does seem that the 'op' theatre will have plenty of work on its hands during the next few days.

Decided to try out the hospital headset for size and hear what they send out. They are not the conventional earphone but a plastic tube which conveys the sound from a control box. Was amazed to hear a Radio Edinburgh programme, or was I hearing things. Couldn't get the headset to stay put as the framework was strained too far apart, so ended up hooking it on my good left ear as my right ear was still out of action.

The Hospital information booklet sent to me was very helpful about all the amenities, and the section explaining the uniforms of the Sisters and the nursing staff, as well as the ancillary staff, took a bit of remembering, but as long as I knew the difference between the Ward Sister and the nurses, I couldn't very well make a mistake.

The nurses themselves had a coded system of coloured cap bands, for qualified nurses, student nurses 1st and 2nd year, and pupil nurses 1st and 2nd year. Upon enquiry as to the difference between them, it seems that student nurses finish as SRN ward sisters or staff nurses after qualification, whereas pupil nurses become SEN agency nurses after their exams have been passed successfully, and they are qualified.

I have been given to understand that I shall be 'starved' tomorrow before and after the 'op' so hope today's meals will keep me going long enough, and that I enjoy the meals laid on for me today.

Wandered down to the day room for a look see and to select a book to get interested in, and suddenly heard my name called by a white coated lady, who explained she was to give me some deep breathing exercises to practice in readiness for coming round after the 'op' to clear the anaesthetic. She explained that unless I breathed in and out correctly I would end up with pleurisy, just like the Pope after his illness. It pleased this lady to know that I didn't smoke, as it makes their job so much easier, and she finally perked me up no end by adding that I seemed very fit lung wise.

As there seemed to be no one else wanting my presence I returned to the day room and selected a James Bond book "From Russia With Love". I don't think I've seen the film so didn't know what the plot was about exactly. I got stuck into it straight away determined to read it right through, as normally I'm not a book worm, so it would give me something to take my mind off things. It was while reading the book that I observed a patient being returned on a trolley to bed after his 'op'. I remember seeing him go off an hour ago, so I guess it's not a long job.

It's now 11.20 and though I've been here just two hours, it seems ages ago that I said goodbye to Joyce. My thoughts were interrupted by Charles who informed me that it was roast lamb for dinner which whetted my appetite in anticipation.

Mr G, who is in charge of the ward, called out to Charles, reminding him that I have to be shaved. Thinks! I did have a shave already this morning so there was only one other place requiring to be done. Would it be a nurse that did it? How would I react to my John Thomas being manhandled by soft fingers? My thoughts were again interrupted when Charles appeared through the screens with soap and razor, and got on with the job. He was very skilful at it, and no doubt had plenty of practice on other patients. When all was completed and the soap wiped away, J.T. looked like a skinhead, and I made a joke about it to Charles.

Made myself decent again and carried on reading James Bond with the occasional interruption for a chat here and there with someone going past. Eve has just given me the first national health sickness certificate, which I promptly started to complete, when suddenly looking around towards the dining table, there sat all the able bodied men waiting for grub up.

I hadn't noticed the large heated food trolley that had sneaked past my bed, and now stood waiting to off load its meals. Hastily shoved away

10

the papers and strolled nonchalantly towards the last vacant place and feeling inwardly guilty at not being alert. There were fourteen of us around the table which made a tight squeeze to get in. This was the first opportunity I'd had to survey my fellow bed mates, and wonder what they were in for.

Exactly at twelve noon the nurses commenced dishing out the lunches which had been selected the day before. Each plate had a paper attached showing the food selected and with the persons name. Most of the men were elderly with about four lads about twenty to thirty years old. The roast lamb was delicious and had been dished up with roast potatoes, sprouts and mint sauce, and rice pudding or prunes were dished up for sweet. There are about half a dozen patients who have their meals in bed as they are not allowed up, and about four others were sitting by their beds with trays. Two others were still sleeping off the effects of the anaesthetic, so I guess they'll be hungry when they come round although they won't be eating anything but a sandwich no doubt.

The time was now nearly 12.30 and decided on a lie down with James Bond, and managed nearly an hours read, when an interruption appeared in the shape of two pretty nurses. One a first year and the other a second year pupil who asked if I had been name tagged. One of them made up a plastic wrist band with my name, ward name Traders, my age, consultants name and my hospital number, which was inserted in a waterproof section, clipped it to my left wrist and I was tagged for life. Next came a barrage of questions to complete a large form they proceeded to fill in. I already remember answering similar questions some time ago.

The time now 1.15pm and it was back to James Bond. All is quiet and occasionally a nurse wandered the length of the ward checking the patients were OK.

My blood pressure and temperature were taken just before 2.00pm, and was told in answer to my question, that the BP is taken every 4 hours and temperature once a day. The Senokots haven't worked on me yet, and the nurses constantly ask if my bowels are open. Two patients have been wheeled out to the 'op' theatre during the last half hour, so the staff are still quite busy.

Suddenly realised it's 2.30pm, when the visitors appeared and took their places by the beds of the "old hands". George's friend, who visits him, has just said that there were hailstones at about 12.00, which was news to me as I was oblivious to the "outside world", as there's so much going on that takes ones mind off any activities outside.

The patient nearly opposite my bed has just returned from his 'op' after being away for 1 hour.

I had brought in some tapestry work that Joyce started several years ago, but due to her eyesight going she could not do anymore. Joyce asked if I was taking anything to do into hospital. When she realised I wasn't doing anything specific, she said "you could finish off this vase of flowers tapestry". It was oval and had a white plastic frame included in the kit and loads of wool. Anyway I thought it about time I made a start on it, and sat down by my bed and began sorting out the colours. I made quite a bit of headway and I did not feel at all embarrassed at being seen doing this type of work, and in fact when nurses saw what I was doing they were quite enthusiastic about my efforts. I daresay they'll be checking its progress each day until it's finished.

It was 3.00 and afternoon tea and biscuits have arrived. Good excuse to knock off tapestry work for a bit of a slurp. I feel sad when the tea comes round during this time, as it must make visitors envious if they also feel like a cuppa.

The second patient opposite me has just returned from the theatre, so will be able to study how long they remain "out" before they come round.

Just had a visit by the Chaplain at 4.15pm, from the United Reform Church in Banstead. He was very interested in my tapestry which I was hard at work on when he appeared. I first noticed him going along the other side of the ward, calling at each bed and having a few words after introducing himself.

The sun is streaming through the windows opposite which must make it quite hot on that side of the ward.

BP and pulse taken again at 5.00pm. Another nurse has stopped and admired the tapestry. Her interest lies more in silk embroidery she informed me.

Mr G happened to be passing and seeing me hard at it, suggested he brought in an antique clock he had which wanted looking at. "More in your line", he said. "No thank you, this will keep me occupied enough" I answered. He must have seen my hospital records giving my occupation as clock mechanic.

Another Chaplain appeared, this time he was from the C of E Church at Belmont. He also was very chatty and explained that a small service would be held in the ward on Sunday. When he left, I carried on with the tapestry and was so engrossed that suddenly realising things seemed quiet, looked at the clock and, horrors it was 6.00pm, and looking across towards the meal table saw it had filled up again in my absence.

Had a quick look at the meal time schedule in the hospital booklet which showed it should have been 6.30pm. It did occur to me that if visiting started at 7.00pm it would be cutting things a bit fine to have supper that late. However, it was vegetable soup, followed by fish cakes, peas and chips for me, while others had salads. I even had another fish cake for seconds. For sweet I had bread pudding like some others, while ice cream had been dished out to those remaining. I have realised that the meals I had been given were already selected by previous patients, so it's just as well my tastes were not too fussy.

Back at my bed, the time now 6.30pm and have just noticed the raindrops on the windows. It had been raining and I had not even noticed anything going on outside. Decided to watch a programme on ITV, and sauntered down to the day room, but upon seeing it was showing a BBC programme did not have the nerve to ask if anyone wanted ITV. Upon returning to my bed noticed a bit of a crisis going on with Bill opposite. Haven't found out yet what he is in for, but it's not my complaint. Looks like they're whipping him off to the theatre with a blockage in his tummy, from a snippet of information I heard.

It was suddenly 6.50pm and Joyce appeared at the ward door, and apparently thinking she was too early, turned round and walked out. The nurses called her back and said it was OK to come in. She was rather puffed after a hectic rush over meal preparation at home before dashing out to catch the train. I let her get her breath back before relating the days events. Quite a few visitors turned up and soon there was quite a hubbub of conversation. Joyce did feel that to catch the 6.48pm train like she did to get here early was rather a rush as it meant getting my sons dinner ready early and dashing off as soon as he came home. So we settled on her coming a bit later in future, which meant a shorter visiting time, but as

14

long as she could take it easy getting here, I felt it would be better in the long run.

At about 7.30 I felt the Senokots were at long last about to work and had to excuse myself and dash off to the toilet. Hope no one noticed my hurried exit too much. It seemed that 8.00pm came upon us all to suddenly and five minutes later the bell was rung and group by group the visitors left, and a hush fell on the ward once more.

The tea and coffee trolley appeared soon after and I thought a coffee would go down well for a change, while I carried on with some more tapestry. Made a start on some of the background colour as a relief from picking out the small patches of darker colours, which were becoming a bit of a strain.

At about 9.00pm decided to pack "work" up for the night and trooped off to the bathroom for a wash down, and test the shaver point for workability. Half an hour later had the urge to phone my daughter Christine and tracked down the telephone trolley and wheeled it to the nearest telephone point to plug it in. Had a 10 pence worth of chat to her and then noticed that the night staff were turning back my bed sheets and guessed it was an invite to get into bed.

Bill in the bed opposite has just returned from the "theatre" and has been away for 3 hours, so guess his crisis was quite serious.

Goodnight Folks. Lights out 10.25pm. At midnight, saw my water jug whipped away. My "Nil by Mouth" had begun.

2. Wednesday May 5th

6.00am.   Good morning. Not much ward activity yet, though Bill across from my bed has been receiving lots of attention so he still seems in a crisis of some sort.

Ernie one of the more mobile patients has started pushing the tea trolley down the ward, dishing out tea to other patients. Looks like he's been lumbered with the job while he's still here. (A proper "tea Ern"). Of course he by-passes my bed, and I feel almost like one of the untouchables with the ominous notice above my head to indicate that nothing must pass through my mouth until after the operation.

Have had my blood pressure, temperature and pulse taken, everything seems normal, so there should be no complications.

The sun is shining through my side of the ward on to the faces of my opposite bed mates, and by the look of things they'll need sunglasses when they sit up.

Just introduced myself to Tom in the next bed to my left. He's been here quite a number of times already for internal examinations of his bladder and insides. He's off first for the theatre at about 9.00am, as his won't be such a big job.

While working on the tapestry, Charles popped tomorrows menu in front of me, for my selection, and the breakfast trolley had just been wheeled in and stopped opposite me. What a temptation, all that food staring at me, and my tummy rumbling like a drain and I cannot even have a sniff.

Breakfast time now, 8.00am and all the mobile men at their places chomping away while 3 of us due for 'ops' cast an occasional eye in their direction. Half an hour later I had my bath and slipped into something more "comfortable" for the theatre. A white gown with a big slit up the back, more of a coming out garment really!

A nurse has just asked me if I've been X-rayed here before, and whether I have had my chest X-rayed. Good job I managed to locate the details among the papers I still had, and no doubt they would find them in my records.

I'm the last to be done this morning, and I should be going out at 11.00am. Must stay in bed now and remain germ free and wait for my "pre med" whenever that may be.

It's just gone 9.00 and Tom has just been wheeled out on a trolley for his theatre visit.

A bell started clanging at 9.15 and have just been informed by Charles that it's Wednesdays fire alarm test. Hey ho, it's all go!

The nurses have been methodically working from bed to bed washing the patients who cannot do for themselves and as the screens are removed one by one, the electric floor sweeper whines away under each bed in turn. Just before 10.00am temptation appears in the shape of the tea and coffee trolley and Gladys goes straight passed my bed on seeing my notice.

A young lad called Kirk, who is at the other end of the ward has just wheeled himself passed my bed in his chair, with his leg out straight on a plank of wood. I had a word with him last evening when I borrowed the phone. He has a portable TV and radio, which has been lent to him and as he is confined to bed mostly with a broken leg, it's quite a comfort for him.

Tom has just returned from the theatre having been away just an hour. He looked quite peaceful as he passed me, and seemed to be awake anyway.

A new patient has just been admitted almost opposite and is getting into his hospital 'gear'.

The second patient is on his way to the theatre, but haven't managed to have a word with him yet.

Just had my "pre-med" at 10.30 and feeling quite relaxed.

Prompt at 11.00, the trolley appeared and I was lifted off my bed on to it, and was on my way at last. A final check at the office to confirm my date of birth and who I was, the blue scarf wrapped round my hair or what there is of it, and away to the lifts. In the ante room a further check as to who I was, in case I'd got mixed up with someone else on the way up here. Was beginning to wonder when I would be told to start counting, but they didn't. Just scratched the back of my right hand and then .... nothing. ZZzzzzz.

Came round later that evening and found I had been back in the ward since 1.00pm.

The ache in my tummy region was similar to the one I had when I've held my water for some time, and I thought I hadn't been done yet, and must have thought out aloud because I was reassured everything had gone off fine. I was puzzled by the tubes coming out of my tummy and one protruding from my J.T. which felt aggravating. Also I found I was in pyjamas, though not matching top and bottom and wondered when the white gown was whipped off, and the pyjamas substituted and by whom? In my half awake state, I looked around me and thought I saw that Georges bed was empty and he had gone out without saying cheerio. I seemed rather confused about my surroundings until a nurse told me I had been shifted up one bed and in fact I was in Georges bed space. I must have been pretty well confused still as the evening wore on, because the night staff were now in and preparations for bed were going on around me.

I was settled down for the night, though I had misgivings about the tubes sticking out, as to whether I would roll over during the night and do some mischief. I was told to drink plenty of water which was recorded each time the jug was refilled.

3. Thursday May 6th

During the early hours, I was woken for temperature, pulse and BP check, which seemed to be done every hour. Hope I wasn't causing too much concern for the night nurses. I felt a bit more like exploring and discovered that the tubes leading from my body went into plastic bags on the floor. So these were the "handbags" I had been told about before I came in to hospital. Also suspended above me to one side was a saline drip and a blood drip. The blood drip was going into my left arm and the saline drip joined the tube coming from my J.T. The tube that was taped to my tummy was the "drain" and was intended to drain the blood from within the area of the wound where the stitches were, into one of the bags, and the other from my J.T. allowed my waste water to flow out uncontrolled by myself. The colour of the liquid entering the bag was red with occasional clots of blood which had to be cleared for a free flow.

I had no idea of the time, as my watch was still in the cabinet drawer, and the electric wall clock was hidden from view by the side screen. Much of the activity had been created by nurses attending to patients confined to bed who were having hands and faces washed.

The side screen was suddenly pushed back and lo and behold it was only 5.30am. It was my turn for face and hands to be washed and I felt pretty helpless at first. All was completed by 6.00 when the tea came round, this time by Tom who must have recovered quite quickly.

The time is creeping on, and have just completed my menu for tomorrow, and had the brainwave of making a note of my order, so that I can bring it to mind next day. Anyway my meals today will, no doubt be had in bed.

20

The day nurses have assembled in the office to discuss their orders for the day, and no doubt be briefed on individual patients progress.

The breakfast trolley has just arrived at 7.50 and there are only 8 men at the table this time. I had cornflakes, boiled egg, bread and marmalade, which went down very well, though I could have done with a bit more. Once the meal was over and plates, etc. cleared away, it was then preparations for doctors rounds at 9.00, after which I was blanket washed by two nurses, mmm, nice.

The dressings on my tummy were changed to get rid of the gory blood mess that had built up. The nurse remarked how neat the stitched wound was, almost like a built in purse zipped up.

So that my bed could be remade, I was helped into the chair which, encumbered by my 2 "handbags" and drip stand, was not an easy feat even though I was helped by 2 nurses. My feet don't feel so cold and clammy now because I am wearing long white leg stockings which I understand is to help the blood circulation.

The visiting barber has just given me a dry shave with an electric razor but it doesn't feel much different than it did before. It's about time the blades were changed.

It wasn't long before the 10.00 tea and coffee trolley made its rounds, but I said I didn't want either as I must drink plenty of water. I had not realised that the coffee and tea consumed was added to my liquid intake, so I learned by my mistake.

At about 11.00, Charles was having a chat with me, and said that when I returned from the 'op' about 1.00pm, yesterday, I was chatting away to him about a variety of subjects, but could not remember anything about it. Then I remembered what George had told me about his wife's visit when he had "come round", which he did not remember.

Lunch time (12.00) came and went, the braised beef, peas, sweet corn and creamed potatoes were followed by fruit trifle, and went down very nicely. It's satisfying not having to wash up after meals.

Was advised to lay down for a rest and after some time I felt the urge to work my bowels and called for a commode. It turned out to be a false alarm as I only passed wind.

Back on the bed to continue my rest, I noticed the saline drip had stopped and that a blood clot had appeared and when I called the nurse, it was "action stations" to free the clot and get the tubes clear again.

Mr G worked hard to get things back to normal and meanwhile Joyce had arrived as the visitors were now in. I felt rather upset that this should have happened just as Joyce had arrived. She must have wondered what was happening as 40 minutes had gone before the screens were removed and she was allowed in.

We both had such a lot to talk about but all too soon the bell went and we had to say goodbye. After Joyce had gone, Bob stopped by and had a long chat. He has polio and other complaints, and can only move about the ward in his wheelchair. He seems very cheerful considering what he is going through, and has been having treatment for some time.

Supper time arrived and I had mine at the bedside table, which consisted of soup, egg salad, tomatoes and chips, ending up with apricots and custard.

At about 7.00, decided to get on to the bed and ease my bladder. Mr G had another session at clearing the blood clots which were giving a few problems, but all was soon back to normal, and the nurses cleared me up and I settled down for the night.

I was still being urged to drink plenty of water and realised I was knocking back glass full's without any feeling of sickness. It's just as well I still have tubes in to drain off the liquid that passes through and I don't have to worry about getting out to the toilet.

At long last the lights went out at 10.00pm and the night nurses had been round for a final check up. I hoped I was in for a good nights sleep.

4. Friday May 7th

Another good morning. Was awaken at 5.00am and had blood pressure, temperature and pulse taken. As well as the blood pressure tablets, I have also been given 2 anti-biotic tablets, three times a day, so hope I don't end up taking too many. Tea came along at 6.00am and I sat in my chair to drink it while thinking about my nights disturbed sleep. Don't know why I couldn't sleep, unless it's because I'm so near the lighted end of the ward, where the night nurses sit on the other side of my screen. Anyway I kept dozing off while drinking the tea, so I was not sorry when 8.00 and breakfast loomed up with Rice Krispies, boiled egg, bread, butter and marmalade. It's funny but it's always boiled egg, never scrambled or fried. Though on second thoughts, boiled eggs are more easily served up.

After breakfast, the floor cleaning programme started, when the beds were moved to the centre of the floor and the electric floor sweepers and polishers slid back and forth over the floor, and the beds then moved back into their places ready for the doctors rounds.

I was sitting in my chair dozing, when I felt someone shake me. It was the ward sister, who told me the doctor had been talking to me. I apologised to him for being asleep and hoped he understood. Anyway he was very pleased at the way things were going and said that my tummy tube can come out today. I have still got the saline drip going into me requiring the supporting stand to be ever near the bed.

I was taken to the bathroom by Kathy who had disconnected the saline drip, as it was easier to move about without it. I was washed down from top to toe and powdered by Kathy, and I did not feel embarrassed as I knew it had to be done, and after all she must have done it plenty of times already, so why should I feel bothered. With a clean pair of pyjamas on (another odd top and trouser combination) it was back on the bed for the removal of the first tube.

The nurse explained that it would be painless and that the tube went under my flesh about 4 or 5 inches, so that she would pull it out reasonably quickly and then place a plaster pad over the opening that would soon heal up. It certainly was a relief to be rid of this tube and also the "handbag" that went with it.

The lunch trolley eventually turned up and everyone waited around expectantly wondering what the menu held for them. As for me, I had ordered poached cod in cheese sauce, peas and creamed potatoes, with ice cream and wafers for afters.

Lunch over, and now what shall I do. Started on James Bond again, but kept dozing off. This happened quite a lot until I came to when a nurse suddenly called my name for my blood pressure and temperature to be taken. The nurse must have thought a bit of exercise might wake me up a bit, so she suggested Derek walk the saline drip stand alongside me while I carried my "handbag". What a strange trio as I shuffled down the ward up to the day room doors, where I said hello to Kirk and then back again.

Derek was a psychiatric nurse spending a few days in our ward for experience. He was quite a good looking chap and did some of the nurses chores like taking the temperatures and the blood pressure readings.

The afternoon visitors came and went and I did some more tapestry. The picture is slowly filling up, though I think I shall have to keep at it a lot more if it is to be finished before I leave here.

Supper time came and went. My menu choice being soup, shepherds pie, creamed potatoes and milk pudding. I am still having my meals sitting in the chair by my bed, as I am still lumbered with the saline drip on its stand, plus of course my pet "handbag".

Joyce came just after 7.00pm and had lots to tell me, and also brought my first lot of mail. As usual 8.00 came all too quick and it was goodbye until next time.

Settled down for a spot of reading and by 9.30 felt I'd had enough of James Bond and decided to hop into bed. Lights went out at 10.15pm and I found I was rather restless. Wish I had taken the sleeping tablet I was offered earlier, but it's too late now.

5. Saturday May 8th

Wasn't very happy about the feeling of sickness every time I drank a glass of water and thought maybe a sitting up position may improve things. The saline drip was holding my attention a lot and I suddenly realised it wasn't dripping and called the night nurse Norma. She gave me a ticking off saying, it's her job to attend to the drip, you should be getting to sleep. I felt like a little boy being put in the corner. It must have done the trick anyway as I did not wake until 5.30.

Tea came round at 6.00 and at 6.30 I was given a bowl of water and told to wash my face and hands, and then settled down to await breakfast time. Time seemed to drag very slowly afterwards and a welcome interruption appeared when I was told the saline drip was to be removed. A final wash out through my J.T. and the saline drip was disconnected, and I was alone with just my "handbag".

Just before lunchtime, Charles informed me I was to have a suppository injection and told to try and hold it for half an hour, as he still isn't happy about my lack of bowel movement. I wondered whether I would hang out until lunch was over, and somehow I did.

One of the nurses asked if I would like a shave and I said she could use my own electric razor, which meant she had to get an extension lead. from the office to plug in near my bed. I did not fancy using the ward razor as it goes from bed to bed and I'm sure must need a new set of blades by now. I did feel a bit more presentable afterwards, which makes a lot of difference to ones moral.

Laid down for the rest period and waited for any signs of the suppository working, but only managed several passes of wind, which at least gave me some relief from the bloated feeling I had.

Before long it was 2.30pm and the visitors started coming in. A nice surprise when I saw Christine (daughter), Jim (son-in-law) and David (son) approaching my bed. I wondered where Steven, (grandson) was, and was told Joyce was walking him around outside in the pushchair.

Everyone wanted to know how the 'op' went, and I explained as best I could leaving out gory details. Christine had the latest pictures of Steven which had been taken at Woolworths and were very good. I called the nurses over to have a look and they drooled over them. It didn't soft soap them enough to let Steven in to see me, however, Joyce eventually came to the ward door. She came to my bed for a quarter of an hour while Jim went out to nurse Steven in the corridor.

When the bell eventually went at 3.30, I did manage to sneak out to the corridor and say "hello" to Steven, who seemed overawed and puzzled by all that was going on. Goodbyes were said all round and off the family went, with Steven still puzzled as to why his Grandad wasn't coming also.

Supper time soon came and went without incident and afterwards I laid down for a while until the 7.00pm visitors started arriving.

Was surprised when my mother-in-law, her son Gordon and his wife Alice suddenly appeared and settled themselves down. They hadn't been here long when Joyce turned up again and gave me some grapes and a get well card. There was so much to relate to a new lot of visitors and Gordon busily tucked into my grapes. He did not require too much coaxing however!

Once again all too soon it was 8.00pm and just as the visitors were leaving, the tea and milk trolley arrived. A chocolate gateau cake was in prominent view and gave the departing guests   a mouth-watering experience.   Joyce seemed to be hanging back a bit hoping for a taste I'm sure.   I was beginning to think it was a Saturday night treat, until told that the relatives of Bill W. had presented it to the ward.   It was shared round the ward and there was still some left over for seconds if anyone wished.

Messed about for the rest of the evening then decided to have a good top wash which made me feel lovely and refreshed. When I emerged from the bathroom, the nurse was "chasing" me to have some attention to the saline drip which had to be re-connected to help clear the bladder as there was still too much blood passing through.

Settled down eventually for the night but not a restful night. Seemed to have an assortment of dreams I vaguely remembered and punctuated by long drawn out blasts of wind, which the night nurse Norma said "kept blowing her off her chair".

6. Sunday May 9th - London Marathon Day

Awoke at 6.00am and seemed to feel a whole lot better, and the welcome cup of tea appeared by one of the new "tea boys". I decided that when that saline drip was removed, and it being Sunday, I would have a close shave and a top wash, and a good brush and comb through my hair.

Thought it about time I had breakfast at the table with the rest of the men. Bob is quite a happy go lucky chap and always cracking the odd joke or two, or passing some comment on something said by one of the other men round the table. Had cornflakes for a change, and the usual boiled egg, bread, butter and marmalade.

Charles seems rather worried about my lack of bowel movement and said I would be given an enema. I had heard about this and of course, wondered what I was about to receive. Things did start happening rather quickly after that and I think Charles was a bit happier.

Mr G then wanted another go at clearing out my bladder, as it still seems the wrong colour. I didn't seem to feel the same pain as before when he emptied the syringe full of liquid into my bladder and then sucked it out in jerky movements until several blood clots appeared. He wasn't too happy when I told him that small ball like clusters had appeared in my back passage, and told me they were piles and that no doubt they had been brought down by the enema. I had heard of this complaint, and wondered if I was lumbered with something else. I was assured they should go back to normal eventually.

After a good bit of washing down and powdering by my nurse Kathy, it was 10.00am and time for a cup of tea.

Kathy suggested I venture out to the fish pond and get some fresh air. It was so good to feel the sun on my face, even though I couldn't strip off like I would have done at home. After a while noticed some activity outside about finding the way of getting the fountain going. No hidden tap could be found hidden among the plants and weeds, and the nearest we got was locating a junction connector feeding the pump.

Hadn't been back inside long before a glass of water was pressed into my hand, and I remembered must "carry on drinking". Anyway I settled back in my chair and knocked back 3 glasses remaining in the jug, then started on another.

The tapestry now came in for a bit of attention, which took me up to lunch time. Another nurse seemed interested in how I did it, and showed her a few stitches.

Lunch time was upon us again, and we were honoured by turkey, stuffing, roast potatoes, cabbage and strawberry blancmange for sweet. Because I still have my pet "handbag" I'm at the end of the table as I get more leg room to fit the bag on the floor. Had a good laugh during the meal at the remarks made by Bob. I don't think he ever stops talking.

Had another go at the tapestry after lunch, filling in the odd patches of colour, with a few outside interruptions, and still knocking back plenty of water.

All of a sudden it was 2.00pm and was told beds were to be tidied up, ship shape ready for the visitors who started dribbling in at 2.20. Joyce arrived about 2.30 after walking the whole of Sutton Lane. I was glad I had lots to discuss, and it seems she had quite a lot to relate about incidents that had happened at home, and how David had to cope with them without my advice. Joyce has thought about redesigning our fish pond, so it seems there will be a lot of planning to be worked out at some stage. After the visitors left, had a good session with the tapestry until the arrival of the vicar from the Banstead United Reform Church and the vicar of St Johns of Belmont, who had brought hymn books, which were passed around the ward. Noticed a few able bodies skiving off to the loo. As it was still near enough Easter, the vicar selected a hymn suitable for the occasion and we all put as much effort into the singing as could be mustered. After a reading from the bible, and a couple of prayers it was all over by 4.30. The two vicars then came by each bed and gave out their local spiritual paper and wished us well.

Supper was started at 6.00pm and was a real riot. Apples were dished out to patients who had ordered oranges. Bob said "show the chef what oranges look like next time".

Two more admissions came in after supper and some more are expected by the amount of activity around the vacant beds, so it looks like being a busy day tomorrow.

Had a go at the tapestry again, but couldn't seem to concentrate and kept making mistakes, so decided to call it a day after the visitors had left. Unfortunately when they trickled in at 7.00pm no one paid much attention and I lost interest in the general hubbub around me.

Decided on a wash down about 7.30. It wasn't until I returned to my bed I suddenly realised the visitors were still here. It's a good thing my bed is at the beginning of the ward. I apologised to sister Sheila, who was sitting with a group of nurses, and think I overheard her say "I've got a soft spot for him", but couldn't believe she was referring to me. I wonder what the 'spot' was anyway.

The patient next to me, who had just moved in, had been to St Helier's previously for an emergency 'op' and was sent home again to wait to be called in again. I had been chatting to him about his trouble which turned out to be the same as mine, though his op will be performed through the penis instead of an incision in the tummy. Having found out enough to satisfy my curiosity I busied myself with some writing, and when I looked over to Bills bed he was reading his bible and I thought, oh well, I've got a bible puncher as a bed mate.

I returned to my writing and suddenly a voice started singing "Jesus wants me for a sunbeam" and then trailed off. I daren't look round in case I was expected to join in. Maybe it was only Bob exercising his voice, after all. It seems that Bill already knew some of the faces here as he had been in this ward previously for examinations.

The night staff started coming in, so there will be change of faces. The lights went out about 10.20pm and then there seemed to be half of hour of noisy comings and goings before things settled down.

Got the last jug of water finished off by 11.30, ready for a new start at midnight.

7.   Monday May 10th

Seems another fine day is about to start, with the usual round of blood pressure, temperature, pulse and pills, followed by our cup of tea, then laze around until 7.00 when it was time for a good wash and shave.

Today was another special one as the final tube, the catheter was to be removed.

After breakfast, I was up on my bed ready for the staff nurse Linda W. to start operations. It was an eye opener to witness the precautions taken for sterility.   One of the assistant nurses is the "dirty" nurse and is responsible for the initial opening of packages and containers.   The "clean" nurse (Linda) stands with hands stuck up in the air, until the surgical gloves are slipped on, then proceeds to sort out her tweezers, cotton wool dabs and the sterile paper cloth which she places over my tummy area with instructions to me not to touch it on any account, so I put my hands above my head out of temptation.

The bladder was washed out first by a series of syringe injections of some liquid until Linda was satisfied that there were no blood clots left. I had been told previously that the tube was held in place by an inflated "bulb", and so I was very interested in seeing this bulb when it came out with the tube. A syringe was fitted to the special outlet and the liquid in the bulb was sucked out. A steady pull on the tube and it was out.   It amazed me how they inserted it in the first place.   Boy, what a relief to be rid of this tubing and the plastic bag. I could now walk about with out my "doggy" going walkies as well.

Linda gave me a clean pair of pyjama bottoms which had to be changed for a smaller pair, as these must have belonged to Fred Emney, and went round me twice. My new instructions were to monitor every drop of water I passed, so now have a "pet" plastic bottle covered with a paper bag to carry to the toilet. The next problem was my daily motions and as they haven't been so good lately, I must have suppositories inserted which will take about an hour to work.

Charles has just given me a part used bottle of Ribena left over by a patient. This will be a pleasant change from plain water.

The 10.00 tea and coffee break has arrived though they are 10 minutes late, due to the busy session this morning. Several more admissions must have come in while I was having the catheter out.

I felt a bit anxious about my bowel movements which didn't materialise on my next visit to the toilet. Things were made worse when I suddenly felt a backache come on which I could not account for other than it may be connected with my kidneys.

Mentioned the pain to Mr G and he prescribed a couple of Panadol tablets for a pain killer. It is very comforting to know that all the activity going on around was similar to the picture a week ago when I was the star attraction.

Just heard a snippet of conversation wafting past that an appendix operation is due in.

Its some time now since I had the suppositories and nothing has worked yet, so Linda has mixed me up a special cocktail to be taken by mouth. It tasted very nice and in other circumstances would have liked another but one of the ingredients in it was crushed up Senokots.

Started on some more tapestry to take my mind off things, and eventually lunch time arrived. Tried to think of what I had ordered. Seem to remember chicken pie or something. More jokes round the table by the "resident comic" to brighten up the new patients.

After lunch decided on a bit of a rest on the bed for an hour or so, then an hour of tapestry "therapy" brought the time round to the blood pressure, temperature and pulse rate crews visit.

The visitors "marathon" started at 2.20 and I was not expecting any visitors myself, so hoped my bowels would soon start operating. Had another go at the flowers on the tapestry with occasional visits to the loo for water samples, but no improvement on the bowel situation.

Suddenly decided at 5.00pm how my whiskers had grown again so got the electric shaver out and trotted off to the bathroom. Decided while there to have a foot bath as they were feeling cold and sweaty. Must get a pair of socks to wear to keep my feet warm.

Just got back to my bed when it was "Gentlemen, please take your places" time and 6.00. Got through soup, ham salad and pear jelly and hoped it would help my bowels. A visit to the loo brought a burst of wind, and break through, not a lot, but a start anyway, which was a relief just before visitors started arriving at 6.50.

Joyce arrived at 7.30 in rather a puffed state which made me feel sad at putting all this exertion on to her. She was pleased that all my extensions and bits and pieces were no longer needed, and she knew I felt happier too. We had a good laugh over the fact that our friend Gwen had sent a get well card which was identical to the one Joyce had given me. Joyce was pleased at my tapestry efforts and will be even more so when it is finished which could be any day.

The visitors bell rang all too soon, especially as Joyce arrived late. Anyway, I walked out to the corridor with her for a final goodnight kiss. Met

Kathy and Sue on the way, two very dedicated nurses, and had a quick chat, before waving my goodbyes to Joyce, who seemed much happier now. Hope she soon starts sleeping better.

Drinks came round soon after and when I had my cuppa, settled down for a session of tapestry. I needn't have bothered as I made a mistake in 2 rows and ended up pulling out 3 rows. That was it, pack up for the night, and it's only 9.15pm.

Had a top wash down for freshness and climbed into bed with 007 again, until my sleeping pill took effect. Had to remember that my water works were under my own control now, so hoped I would not disgrace myself or the bed. The night nurse Millie said she'd smack my bum if I did. Ooh- er! By 10.20 the lights were out. Goodnight.

8. Tuesday May 11th

Another sunny morning. I certainly had a good nights sleep and only got out of bed once at 2.45 to fill my bottle for checking, then back to sleep again till nearly 6.00am when the tea came round.

Had the usual round of pills and blood pressure, etc. A bit of excitement to break the monotony, when one of the hospital porters came through the ward chatting with the staff. It seems this porter took part in the London Marathon and on his way past my bed just had to call him over and congratulate him and gloss over his medal.

Read the final exciting episode coming up in the James Bond book, and then it was 7.00am and time to think about a wash down. My bowel movement is still not forthcoming, which is very annoying, especially when the nurse asks me how my bowels are.

Suddenly noticed it was nearly 8.00 and horrors! when I returned to the ward the men were already eating, and I'd done it again. There wasn't even a gap to slip into, until someone squeezed up for me. Anyway, it was only 7.55 so I wasn't really late.

Didn't have time to look up my list of what I'd ordered so started on cornflakes, then halfway through remembered I'd put down for porridge, then thought, oh well a bit of roughage won't hurt. Finished off breakfast with boiled egg, bap roll, butter and marmalade and 2 cups of tea, and back by my bed in time for doctors rounds at 8.30.

Was told by the doctor that stitches should come out tomorrow. I showed great happiness on my face which I'm sure reflects the results of their hard work.

Just finished the final chapter of James Bond book, and felt sad that they got him in the end. The urge to go to the toilet had slowly been building up with a pain in my tummy and I got to the toilet with the faint suspicion that this was it. Soon as I sat down and got my bottle placed in position, - whoosh, it was out and all pains gone - just like that. Charles will be pleased when I tell him.

Had a wander outside to the fish pond, but though it was gorgeous being in the sun, there was still a stiff breeze, so decided to return indoors. As I made my way back to my bed, I had a natter with one or two of the blokes and really felt on top of the world.

Seeing the bod in the bed opposite me using the phone, gave me the thought to ring Christine when he'd finished. Was I annoyed when the nurses descended on his bed and whipped the screens around him, so now I couldn't see when he had finished his call. After an interval, called Cathy, the Irish nurse over to peep in and see if the phone was free. It was, so she kindly wheeled it over to me. Got through to Christine and had a nice long chat, as I had lots of things to talk about. The only trouble was the "jaws" of this "bandit" grabbed 20p of my change before I decided to call a halt, before it all ran out. The post has just arrived and there was a comic get well card from my mother-in-law. The tea and coffee trolley had also arrived, as I wheeled the phone trolley back to its "stable", and decided on coffee instead of tea for a change.

Joyce apparently won't be in to see me today, as she is staying at Christine's overnight, baby sitting, and will be going on to work from there next morning. Christine and Jim will be bowling, so only hope Steven does not play up too much. Must remember to phone Joyce later this evening.

Another burst of bowel movement was upon me and I feel it is improving each time. It's aggravating having to keep filling my bottle for my water check.

A nurse has just requested that I hop on my bed for the removal of the plaster over my stitches. A steady pull and it was peeled off to reveal a neat row of stitches. Even the small hole that the drain tube came out from has closed to almost nothing. Well done, doctors and staff.

Mentioned to the nurse that I felt like a bath, but she advised me to wait until the doctor had seen the stitches this afternoon. Had to make do with a wash down top and bottom.

The operating theatre seems to have been busy this morning. Three bods have gone off that I know of.

Have been told by the nurse to improve on my water intake and to get at least 3 litres of liquid down me by 7.00pm, to improve the colour of my bottle samples which at the moment are a shade of brown, which would put Jim off beer for life, I reckon.

Just found out there's another "Les" in the ward. Apparently Bob had called out "Les" to someone, and I answered at the same time as another chap. It seems that Bob wanted me to call Barry, who is in the side ward, for lunch, but Barry told me he would be having it in bed as he has just had some painkiller injection and wasn't up to it.

As there's a few minutes to go before the 'off' for lunch, have done my good deed and put all the chairs round the table.

The old chap in the first bed opposite has returned from St Helier Hospital where he had some tests or something.

The call for "Gentlemen, please take your places" from Charles was eventually heard and the table soon filled up with hungry faces. Steak pie, vegetables and carrots, followed by stewed apples and custard was the menu for today. The smell of food must have been too much for Barry in the side ward, as he suddenly appeared at the table soon after we had started eating. He managed to squeeze in beside me, and when I say squeezed, it certainly was a tight one as he is a bit on the stouter side than myself. From conversation that got going, we learnt that he's a DJ on a radio station and has had scores of get well cards sent to him from his listeners.

The theatre op patients that returned could not have been too serious, as they are awake and sitting up in bed.

After lunch decided to get a few rows of tapestry done, then lay down for an hour and listened to Gloria Hunniford's programme, only to be interrupted for temperature, blood pressure and pulse to be taken.

In no time at all, it was time for the daily troop of visitors to start, but thought I better nip off to the toilet to feel a bit more comfortable, especially as I felt wet down below for some reason. Tidied up my hair, even though no one was visiting me, and was prepared to smile when necessary. Got my tapestry out, as it seems to attract conversation from interested visitors when passing. At 2.25pm the visitors arrived.

Sheila, the ward sister, seeing I had no visitors after half an hour seized the opportunity to explain what my operation had entailed. It was very interesting and matter of fact, and she answered my intimate questions with out any gory details.

Afternoon tea arrived at 3.00pm and I ended up with 2 cups, as it all helps with my liquid intake. Not so many visitors this afternoon, as I stared about me in between plugging away at the tapestry,

41

when the bell tinkled at 3.33pm and all was back to normal.

After 4.00, I sorted out a clean towel, my washing and shaving gear and trotted off to my favourite bathroom, which also had 4 sink units, so we can muck in and chat while we wash, while we shave, while we ....., etc. etc.

As I cannot have a proper bath yet because of my stitches, I started top most and when completed and powdered, etc. had a brainwave to sit on the bath board to do my feet and legs up to my operation. The water was glorious and the feeling of serenity glowed throughout. Incidentally the bathrooms and toilets have engaged tabs, but anyone can walk in if you're at the sink or in the bath. I had my back to the door anyway, so was not too worried. Even the nurses pop their head round the door if they are looking for anybody or checking the room. My wash down was followed by a close shave, and I really got down to those bristles. Another thought crossed my mind. How about a hair wash? There was a hospital bottle of shampoo on the shelf and having filled the sink with water, I had an hour with Maison Leslie. My hair certainly was the better for it, and I was feeling great and pleased with myself for accomplishing so much. With a matching top and bottom pair of pyjamas for a change, I emerged from the bathroom looking less like a clown.

As soon as I appeared, nurses flustered round me saying "where have you been? We've been looking for you for the last half hour." I explained my activities and was amazed when I realised it had taken me a whole hour, and I still hadn't combed my hair. It seems I was not by my bed for the ritual temperature, pulse and blood pressure to be taken, and no one knew where I'd gone. I said to Kathy, "you should have looked in the bathroom first". I had told my bed mate where I was going, and he even came in the bathroom at first to study some stain on his leg.

Anyway, I wasn't scolded too much and they got on with the temperature and blood pressure checks. It was while Kathy was taking my blood pressure, that I said to her, "I've been suspicious of you", and went on to outline the fact that she leaves here late, yet still arrives looking so fresh and on time the next morning. Then I said "I think you are a robot, and if I peeled back your skin, I'd find a lot of electronics underneath". I told Kathy I had a gadget that tests for robots and produced my pocket metal detector and ran it cursory over her body and made sure the red lamp glowed occasionally. She guessed, of course, I was fooling and had a good laugh about it.

After tidying my hair, I had a session with my 'bottle', which was very satisfactory as it was getting paler each time. My water intake must be doing the trick.

The 6.00pm dinner call eventually came, and I settled back at the table to await the soup, poached plaice, mushroom sauce, peas and chips. Unfortunately I had to be content with cod, though I did have much trouble with the bones. Finished the meal with a banana.

Remembered to phone Joyce, who was at Christine's, after 7.00pm, so called in to Barry's room to collect the trolley, and got through to a very upset Joyce. It seems Steven, my grandson, would not settle down, and she was getting rather tired. I was nearly in tears for her, knowing what she was going through. My 10 pence call must have only been halfway through when the line was cut off. Fed in 5 pence to check the coin slot but still nothing. Anyhow dialled again, and Joyce came on, having guessed I was cut off. Managed to convince

Joyce all was well with me and it was all systems go. Said goodnight and hoped she would have a settled night sleep, once Christine and Jim were back in command.

The tapestry has now been reduced to 25 rows, so all things being well, it should be finished in time. Had a word with Kathy to find a pair of socks as my feet seemed cold even in my slippers, until Joyce brought me some socks on Wednesday. The only thing available was the tubiflex bandage, and Kathy's idea of cutting a couple of lengths which just slip over my feet, worked beautifully.

Had another dig about Kathy being a robot. I had heard Kathy talking to a patient who had just come round from his op. He must have asked her what year it was, as Kathy replied it's 2001. I reminded her of this and said "you gave yourself away just now, when you said the year was 2001". She has such a lovely chuckle.

The night staff have already come on, and one of them is an agency nurse. The other one Millie, must have had some dental treatment during the day, as she's not too happy about things. Kathy and her helping hand, Judy, have finished for the night and have gone home.

It's now 9.15 and went to the loo for a final bottle specimen before taking my sleeping pill and settling myself in bed for a relaxing listen to the radio and a bit of tapestry. Lights went out 10.30pm - Goodnight.

9. Wednesday May 12th

Good morning! Awoke at 6.00am, with sun beginning to show through the windows. Usual temperature, pulse and blood pressure routine completed. The tea trolley has just been wheeled through to the other end of the ward and a volunteer called for to do the pouring out. No doubt I would have been lumbered with the chore had it stopped at my end. Anyway it may be my turn tomorrow.

Washed down my anti-biotic and blood pressure tablets when my cup of tea arrived. Decided for a change I would have a second cup to increase my liquid intake, but would have to get my skates on before the tea wagon ran dry. The tea pot, an aluminium one was massive and must have been still half full or half empty, and when I lifted it, the weight surprised me.

Will have to get some weight training exercises in today to have my right arm in condition. Come to that I shall have to get both arms into shape as the urn has two handles.

The time is creeping up to 7.00am and I am noting the beds that have NIL BY MOUTH cards above them indicating the patients due for ops.

My bed mate Bill, is on the 'op' menu today and is gradually preparing himself for the ordeal, had his bath and donned the white gown with the split down the back. Bills operation is also for a prostatectomy but he is uncertain if his will be an incision like mine or by probe, which sounds painful.

Now 8.00 and the whiff of food assails the ward. Hard luck on the nil by mouth bods, whose absence makes the table a bit empty this morning. Porridge, bacon and egg, bread, butter and marmalade went down very well, amid lots of discussion among other things, home decorating. Leading up to the new idea of "contour" wall covering, which is one scheme I used in my kitchen. Was able therefore to share my experiences of hanging this covering which looks just like tiles.

Was busy chatting to a couple of bods about 'ops' when I suddenly noticed lots of activity about my bed, and found it was to be shunted down the ward 5 bed spaces. It was almost a case of take up thy bed and walk, only this time it was wheeled. The bed locker also accompanied the bed, much to my annoyance as the drawer was a sticky one, I always had a job to pull open, so would have relished a change.

Had a check on the radio socket for workability and laid out my cards again, and suddenly realised Mr B was on his rounds being 8.45am. When Mr B and his retinue approached my bed, I automatically stood up which normally no other patients did. He was very pleased with my progress and said that the stitches may come out tomorrow, Thursday and I might be out by the weekend.

I must say here, that everything that goes on in the ward is like a well oiled piece of machinery, and the planning that goes on before hand must be precise. Anyway I'm off the measuring bottle to tabulate my water output and also my water intake need not be recorded anymore.

The blokes due for 'ops' are having their screens pulled round one by one in readiness for the pre-med, so I guess by 9.00am the first one, my old bed mate Bill, who is now in my old position number 1 bed, will be on his way. I shall look forward to his return and be able to reflect how I may have reacted when I returned to the ward.

Have just spotted the theatre trolley standing by to take Bill off, so thought I'd sneak away to the toilet unencumbered by my bottle, and hung about while the orderlies and staff nurse double checked his name tag, and put the blue head cover on him. Managed to wish him a speedy return as he 'sailed' by.

Upon reaching my bed, I noticed the lady that deals with the mail approaching and goody she had something for me. It was a get well card from Christine, and I had to laugh when I saw the picture. I had to show it to Eve, the mail lady, and convince her I wouldn't be leaving the hospital that way. It showed two beds, and in one a patient was making cane baskets, while the other bed now unoccupied had a 'rope' ladder made of canes tied to the bed, and leading out of the window. Christine had added the words inside the card, "Hope you escape soon".

Managed to get to the phone and thank Christine for her card which had really bucked me up, and tell her my news. Steven, my grandson, was grizzling in the background and Christine said Joyce had got off to work alright and that Steven had eventually got to sleep by 9.00pm last night and had woken at 7.30 this morning.

The weekly Wednesday fire alarm test has just gone off, so I guess all systems are go. Wonder what would happen if there was a fire anywhere.

The senior nurse has just pulled the screens round me, so that my "wound" can be inspected. "It's coming on nicely", she said, but my stitches might not be out tomorrow after all.

The senior nurse, never found out her Christian name, though her initials were J.E., went off to get my bath ready, but came back because it was engaged. She suggested I wait till after coffee.

Just had a chat with my near neighbour at number 3 bed, who is having his daily walk. He's awaiting a prostatectomy and hernia op, but his blood pressure is too high at present. He has his 'pet' he takes walkies with him.

Had a chat with another couple of 'cases' who just strolled by. One of them, the DJ (already mentioned) Barry, had a hernia op and is still in the side ward which he says he prefers as it is so airy. The other chap was in for a stone removal but though he's been on plenty of water, he cannot pass it. He's leaving today and says he feels such a fraud having been here since last Friday and nothing achieved.

Approaching 10.00am and it's coffee time, so will just stretch my legs a little, and collect my drink. Bill has not yet returned, so will see about my bath. I wallowed in freedom for the first time since last Wednesday and weighed myself in my skin at 56.3 kgs.

Returning to the ward eventually spotted my friend Bill back in his bed at number 1, and seemingly awake. I asked Kathy if I could speak to him, she said "yes, but not for long as he's resting". He was pleased to see me and I welcomed him back. Have noticed the constant attention paid to him while he's resting and the monitoring of his pulse, etc. until the nurses are satisfied they can leave him to come round normally on his own.

During my conflabs with other able bodied patients I learnt that a lad of about 20, Tom, has been here since yesterday and is due for a wisdom tooth 'op'. I sat next to him yesterday and have only been on nodding terms with him so far. He seemed very quiet and I expect very scared. I wish I could have encouraged him to relax into the very capable hands he'll be in.

Time now creeping up to 11.30am, and soon it will be lunch time. Haven't far to go for the table now my bed has been shifted. Charles' call to the table eventually came at 12.00 for lunch to be served. Roast beef, Yorkshire, roast or creamed potatoes and cauliflower, mmm!

Only seven of us at the table for this sitting, as the rest are confined to their beds. Quite a young lad has been admitted who is sitting opposite me now. He's not very talkative, of course, and no doubt feeling a bit scared. I saw him earlier today sitting in the day room with his mum and wondered what he may be in for. Couldn't be my complaint at his age. He is two beds down from me, number 7, so I guess I'll soon get chatting to him and put him at his ease.

Three 'op' cases have so far returned, and I lost count of who went and when, the last one just back in place at 12.45.

The lad with the wisdom tooth has just been brought back. Said hello! to the young boy in number 7, his name is Tom, and he's in for treatment to a septic toe. We seem to have a few more Toms in here at the moment.

Having a bit of a lie down for a while, contemplating my navel as they say, and must have dosed for a few minutes or so, when the theatre trolley returned with another patient who was parked opposite my bed. The 'op' theatre certainly has been busy today. This ones the short round face chap, I've noticed around.

Time for blood pressure, pulse and temperature round, 1.30pm. Began to think I was being deserted now that I'm getting better, but I realised, of course, that the 'post op' patients come first now.

The "wisdom tooth" lad has a sort of frame round his chin to give it some support, I suppose. Guess it will affect his eating to some extent.

Just had a session in the toilet, 2.00pm, and it seems my bowel movement has started at last.

Tom at number 7, has an arrow painted on

his right toe towards a rather angry red inflammation near his nail. His stay will not be too long it seems. It is fast approaching visiting time and this is the first day I've been able to study the activity that goes on before the visitors are allowed in. Today with the number of 'ops' completed there has been quite a lot of tidying up to do before the 'off'. Meanwhile you can see the visitors outside the door champing at their bits eager to burst in.

It's just 2.32 and 'they're off'. The same faces appear each time, and now I am further down I can pair off which visitors belong to which patient.

Have noticed that Charles has been sitting by number 1 bed occupied by Bill, no doubt talking to him like he said he was chatting to me when I came back. My mind is still a blank on that period even though Charles said I was talking back to him. Will be able to test it out with Bill when I speak to him eventually after he's recovered fully.

Tea arrival at 3.00pm. Cease embroidery for 5 minutes while I savour a hot cuppa and take a look round. It must be so tantalising to the visitors to have patients drinking tea under their noses when they can't have one.

Bit sharp on the bell today, 3.28, especially as they were late letting them in.

My friend Bill at number 1, has requested the phone and as I have just phoned Joyce with a couple of memos I jotted down, I pushed the trolley up to my old 'pad' and set it all up for him, then went off for a wash and shave when I was sure no one would be wanting me for blood pressure, etc.

It's now 4.45 and normally I've realised, I would be leaving work and making my monotonous daily trek through Guys Hospital grounds on my way to London Bridge station and wondering if the 17.02 from platform 9 would be running. Hey ho! those days will return soon enough, no doubt.

Just had my 5.00pm blood pressure, temperature and pulse taken plus the anti-biotic tablet thrown in. Carried on with the tapestry and found I'm getting on like a house on fire. Decided to tidy up the unholy mess of coloured wool in the bag, and laboriously disentangled each colour and laid them out on the bed before tying each skein separately. Time seemed to fly and it's 5.45 and the others have started assembling at the table. Only 7 of us again sitting, the remainder having regained consciousness were now being waited on by their beds. It was a real laugh at the table with Bobs comments. Two of the men doubling up with laughter enough to open their stitches. The DJ, Barry, complained that too much laughing played up wicked with his hernia 'op'.

After dinner, decided to give the Crossroads serial a miss, because the snooker fanatics will want to switch over at 6.50, so fell back to 20 minutes of tapestry.

The visitors started in at 6.55 and while carrying on with the tapestry, mentally pictured Joyces train leaving Banstead at 7.08pm and rattling along the well worn track on its way to Belmont, where she should arrive by 7.11. Her steps, in my mind, were traced over the footbridge, down the other side and a slow plod up from the ticket office to the main road. I assisted her across the pedestrian crossing (mentally) and then counted up to 500 which should have brought her to the corner opposite the hospital. Saw her safely across the busy road and into the hospital entrance. Up the windy (not gale sort) path to the front entrance, a good push on the front door and then a count down along the corridor and I looked up just as Joyce made her entrance, and homed in on me. Hello darling! We had so much to talk over, the trials she had endured with our grandson Steven, the previous evening were related. Steven certainly knew his Mum wasn't on hand for his usual bit of comfort.

My news for today was very varied, though I was able to say I should be home at the weekend. (Depends on how quick they get fed up with me).

The ward sister Sheila stopped for a chat, and said how happy she was that all had gone so well. I said this is just like a holiday for me, with Joyce adding "yes, he's really enjoying all the fuss taken over him". Sister said, of course, that is what we aim to do, and that I was very well behaved.

Wow, 8.00pm already and there goes the tinkling bell and as Joyce hadn't had the full session decided to have a few more moments together. We walked along the passage and said our goodnights, and I hoped Joyce would not have long to wait at Belmont for her train home.

Hot drinks suddenly made an appearance, and the trolley slowly wound its way down the ward. I had 2 cups of coffee and as I'm not on measured liquids anymore, who cares?

The pulse, temperature and blood pressure nurse is doing her rounds, but she has by passed my bed tonight (nobody loves you baby!).

Technical problem has just cropped up in the bed opposite, as the nurse has been called to check the bed light. I offered to replace the bulb for her from the spare bed lamp next to me, thinking the other one had just blown. Wasn't until I'd swapped the bulbs over that I found the patient hadn't had his wall switch on, and his bulb was OK. The nurse was just going off duty too, so that saved a bit of a panic.

It is now 9.00pm and I shall soon think about settling down for the night. Have just heard a loud statement coming from the TV room, and was just in time to hear that one of our ships had been under attack by Argentinean fighters but had defended itself successfully having blown up 2 jets, the 3rd one whizzed back home.

The pulse, temperature and blood pressure nurse came back to me, so I wasn't missed after all. She also turns back the sheets ready for nipping into bed, and while she was doing the one next to me, I said "no ones using that bed". I suggested maybe my wife could use it as she hadn't had many good nights since I'd been here. The nurse was Chinese and had a chuckle at my suggestion.

Guess I ought to make a move, it's 9.15, and try to get an hour of tapestry done. The Chinese nurse spotted my tapestry and asked if it was mine, and in reply to my affirmative, she added "aren't you clever". Did wonders while sitting in bed doing the tapestry and reached the row just under the flower pot.

The main lights have just gone out, so my own one must soon follow.

Being as I'm still awake and feeling no signs of dropping off and went to the toilet, and on returning to bed, wrote up events to the present time. Bob had his light on till 11.30 and I had been laying with my eyes away from his bed. He writes all his letters at night apparently.

When I first laid down at 10.30pm, he suddenly called across and said "are those your socks hanging on the cupboard, Les?" and to my answer of "yes" he said, "you want to hang them outside the window, the airs fresher." "It took me 2 days to get this pair," I said, "so I don't want them pinched." Bob then related an incident when he walked from Kings Cross to Sutton and arrived home with feet burning and hung his socks out of the window. Next day his wife went past the house on a bus and saw his socks having a good airing, so he had some explaining to do. I found it difficult to hear Bobs every word as normally during the day his voice is deep-booming, and now, he'd toned it down because of the other sleepers and I had my left ear cupped forward to catch every word, to make sure I gave the right answer in response.

I did eventually manage to slide down the bed and have another go at sleeping, but the whirr of the ripple machine under the bed near me created a steady hum. These machines pump air in and out of alternate folds in the under blanket giving a ripple sensation. The night nurse must have been telepathic as she suddenly switched off the one near my bed and once again peace reigned.

Sleep, however, still eluded me, what with the variety of snore tones and heavy breathing, I kept feeling sweaty so stripped off the top of my pyjamas which felt quite damp. It was 2.30am, when I wandered off to the loo with my diary in an attempt to break through in my bowel operation.

Dennis joined me out there and we were chatting about many things. He's having plenty of trouble with his piles apparently.

Got back to bed eventually and tried hard to drop off to sleep. Poured myself a Ribena drink for something to do and must have gone to sleep about 4.00am.

10. Thursday May 13th

Awoke at 5.30, couldn't have slept long, and listened to music and news. The nice Chinese girl was on the pulse, temperature and blood pressure rounds. Shoved my pyjama top back on and noted that my blood pressure was much lower than it had been of late - whoopee.

Spotted the tea trolley being wheeled in so got my socks and dressing gown on in readiness for my chore. That teapot was certainly heavy and required two hands to lift it. Filled up half a dozen cups and sugared them to the individual requirements and gradually worked my way down the ward. Suddenly realised I hadn't been using the tea strainer, which must be rectified before I get to the "old hands". Was getting a bit worried that the pot was getting lighter, and emptier and I had a return trip to make for refills.

What do I do about topping up. I then learned that there was a big jug of hot water under the trolley plus more tea and milk. No one explained this when I took over the "shop". So in with the water and half a dozen spoonfuls of tea, a good stir and I was in business again. Had to remember to grab my own two cupfuls before the whole lot went. It made me feel proud to be able to carry out this duty which seemed an important cog in the machinery of the hospital, and I felt happy about the encouragement from everyone.

Eventually I went round collecting up the empties and stowing them on the trolley ready for its removal, and that was the end of my first day as 'char' wallah. (The RAF slang for 'tea boy').

Charles came on duty at 7.25 and did his round of dishing out the menus for tomorrows selection. This was my signal to get my ablutions complete and standby for breakfast. Managed to get to a wash basin by 7.30 and suddenly realised I'd been on the go since 6.00am.

Had a chat with a young lad who had three wisdom teeth removed. His left cheek is swollen quite a lot, so things are rather painful for him. His name is Tom also, so that makes 3 in the ward that I know of.

However, ablutions now complete and it was back to my pad, and all seated at the breakfast table by 7.50, for porridge, boiled egg, roll and butter, marmalade and tea. The sun feels lovely and warm on my back while having breakfast, so it seems like being a hot day.

Was sorting out my cabinet drawer when Bob across the way spotted an envelope I had, and asked if I was in touch with the Philatelic Bureau. This lead to a new line in conversation and we discussed at long length our interests and hobbies. He was interested in the phone system I once had before I moved to Banstead, and seemed enthusiastic about the description of my son David's' railway items he has collected.

Must have been gassing to Bob for quite a while when he nudged me saying "I'd better get back to my bed, as Mr B and company were only 2 beds away from mine. When my turn came, I stood up smartly (why I don't know) and the doctor remarked "what a sprightly young man" (honestly I can't do a thing wrong). He was told I would be going home on Saturday and hoped I'd enjoy today's lovely sunshine.

When the ward settled down to its normal routine I was idly looking at the NIL BY MOUTH notices above some of the beds (remembering when they had applied to me) and suddenly had an idea. An anagram was worked out from the letters and in no time had come up with "I'M HUNY BOLT". I was thrilled, and set to work on a blank space of one of

56

my "get well" cards and painstakingly pencilled in the letters. Will have to ask the ward sister if I can display it over my bed, hope she says yes.

It's coming up to 9.45 and will soon be coffee time, so poured myself a Ribena drink, and sauntered out to the day room, and spotted the gardeners mowing and tidying up the grounds around the fish pond. Thought here's my chance to find out about the water pump, and luckily I spoke to the chap who had actually installed it. He rather deflated my ego by telling me that the fountain won't be on for 2 weeks, as they have such a lot of work on around about, and the pond must be cleared out before they get the pump going. I told him I'll be back to see it working during one of my outpatient visits.

As it was not all that warm in the sun decided to return to the ward where I found the coffee trolley had arrived 10 minutes early, so it will help to wash my Ribena down.

The barbers doing his rounds again, but I'll not trouble him for his services. Just "overheard" the barber say in a loud voice, four beds away, "you can give me a tip, but you don't have to pay anything".

One of the elderly gents at the beginning of the ward has just returned from an outing to his flat, where he was taken earlier to find out if he can negotiate any steps or obstacles when he is finally left on his own. It hasn't escaped my notice the assistance he's been given at odd times and have been puzzled at the various plaster casts, leg shaped, that have been past my gaze. It seems they are working on some form of general support.

It is now 10.30 and there is an air of laxness now that all the doctors questions and investigations have ended. Will nip out to the loo now and hope to jog the sisters' mind that I wanted a word with her.

Wandered out to the pond again as the sun was so inviting, sorely tempted to strip off like Bob has. Still hadn't pinned sister down to ask her yet, and when Charles came out to speak to Bob I thought - who better to ask, so I drifted about until I saw he was about to come in, and showed him the card with "I'M HUNY BOLT" printed on it. He laughed when I explained its meaning and said he didn't think sister would mind if I put it above my bed.

I had to come to Charles rescue again when he asked me what was on the menu today, and my note book was consulted. The notice is now stuck up above my head and sister is approaching with my pills. She gazed at the notice and said "I don't know what that means", and I replied there's only 3 people so far that do. She wanted to know why I wanted to speak to her, and what was my problem. Pointing to the notice, I said it was a point of etiquette I asked her first if I could put it up. I just had to tell her what it meant, and she thought it very ingenious. I also cleared up a clinical point regarding my 'op' again, and then mentioned that I'd heard on the "grapevine" she was getting married.

The vicar last Sunday mentioned it when he said one of the nurses on the ward would be getting married at Belmont. Anyway sister said it is not till next April, when she can get her Mother over from New Zealand. Now there's another snippet I'd learned, she's a Kiwi, a real Sheila.

Have just had my temperature and blood pressure taken by Karen, who was very intrigued by my board above the bed. I made her work it out by suggesting she's been hanging them up all week, and it's an anagram. Then she got it.

As it was nearly lunch time, I nipped out into the sun again and played around with the goldfish in the pond until called for lunch. Only 8 of us sitting down this time, to Chicken garni, creamed spuds, omelette, beans, followed by rhubarb and custard. It was as usual, a laugh a minute with Bob and crowd, egged on by Barry.

The nurses were bunched around my bed studying the anagram notice above my bed, and attempting to decipher it. A few of the brainy young men round the table got it and eventually everyone knew. It gave a bit of extra excitement anyway.

I phoned Joyce after lunch and caught her at work in case I couldn't fit it in later. My free and easy approach to life rather upset her especially as she hadn't had a good morning. I confirmed that I would not be out until Saturday, and my stitches would be taken out on Friday.

Sat outside in the sun with my sleeves up until 2.00pm with Bob, who had been cracking endless jokes and wise cracks with all and sundry that went by.

I was delighted when Bob asked if I would get him an orange squash, and my personal attention was appreciated especially as he can only get around in a wheelchair, and with his large bulk, he's all heart and soul.

Earlier when I went outside, Kirk, the lad with the broken leg was sunbathing in his wheelchair with his leg stuck out horizontally with nothing on but a towel loosely across his middle. He's always "equipped" in sunbathing 'gear' because he wears nothing while in bed and has to stay in bed for meals and only gets up for trips to the bathroom and toilet and only partly covers up on route. Anyway the nurse called Caroline who is in charge of him while he's out here, asked the ward sister Sheila for permission to take Kirk in his chair around the grounds. She returned from sister with permission to go and a dozen do's and don'ts to obey. My request to sister, to go with them was refused however, very sweetly, by explaining that as I still have my stitches in, if an accident occurred away from the ward, they would be responsible. So I resigned to remain with Bob soaking up the sun from waist up while I was only uncovered up to the upper arm.

The appearance of Bob's nurse indicated that it was temperature and blood pressure time. She poked his personal thermometer into his mouth to stop him talking (which it didn't do anyway) while she got on with his pulse taking. Bobs other hand idly slipped down her legs, which she promptly discouraged in a firm way. His thermometer looked as if he'd snapped it off, as there was only about an inch showing. Talk about a north and south. Then my nurse appeared with my thermometer and blood pressure gauge, and under Bobs constant quips was in a proper fit of giggles and had to control myself, so that a correct reading could be obtained. Luckily all readings were normal as was my blood pressure.

The visitors arrived at 2.30 and as there were none for me, decided to gather up my tapestry work and go outside in the glorious sun. Bob was already out there with his wife chatting away merrily. Stretched myself out on the long seat with my sleeves rolled up and got down to serious work. Was oblivious to things going on around me until I heard that tea and biscuits were on their way round. Gwen the tea lady served it to Bob and I through the open window of the day room. As I had done nearly 3 rows of the tapestry decided I'd had enough, and chatted with Bob and his wife. It appears she locked herself out of her house this morning, when phoning Bob, and the next door neighbour had to endeavour to let her in again. She and Bob have apparently had their share of troubles one way and another, and it seems that lately their car has caused them much worry and expense, for new parts. They have 3 married daughters and 6 grandchildren between them, which make my one little grandson, Steven, a lone beginner. The chat seemed to cover everything, even railway fares and transport in general.

All too soon the visiting hour was over and I wandered back to my bed and thought out my next move. Christopher in the bed opposite had been thinking up an alternative anagram for my bed, and between us eventually came up with "YOUTH'N LIMB" which I thought was better than my first effort. This was now printed out neatly and stuck up in place of the other one.

Barry asked for a list of nurses names, staff and patients, he could read out on Sunday during his 2.00 - 5.00pm programme on the JFM radio show. I shall be looking forward to hearing him and his patter.

Had a shave about 5.00 and used my new Bic razor. Unfortunately when I use a new razor I end up with a few nicks. This time was no exception and I ended up walking about with tufts of cotton wool around my chin, which I must remember to remove before Joyce comes to see me.

Young Tommy came back from his op at 5.20 and is still asleep with his legs under a frame leaving his feet free. Apparently he kicked his toe through a glass door. Bob came up with his immediate wit, saying "I bet that pained him" and even something funnier, which I cannot remember.

Supper time was suddenly upon us and 9 able bodied patients sat up to dine. Had soup, sardine sandwich and an offer from Charles as going spare. Finished off 2 fruit trifles for my sweet and that was that. The supper didn't go with the usual amount of ribbing and joking by Bob and others present, so guess other things were on our minds. There are 5 empty beds so may be it will be a bit quiet tonight.

It's 5 minutes to seven and the visitors are arriving. Suddenly noticed lots of activity around Bills bed at number 1, when the screens were thrown round his bed and the nurses brought in a saline drip stand. Joyce arrived at 7.20, all hot and bothered with my camera, and wondered why I wanted it. I really felt miserable knowing how tired she must be making this journey to visit me, but she didn't want to disappoint me. Time slipped by and 8.00 came with no sign of the bell sounding. The visitors were voluntarily leaving on their own, when the bell eventually tinkled at 8.05. I walked Joyce to our departure point and said our goodnights, and with a sad heart, watched her go through the exit door, knowing how miserable she must be feeling, wending her way home on her own in her tired state.

Returned to my bed and tidied my drawer and reorganised the papers, I wanted to work on. Went round the ward getting the names of the patients and some nurses to complete Barry's list for his radio programme due this coming Sunday, and passed it over to him and let him sort it out.

An urge to put the head phones on suddenly hit me and I heard a girl called Theresa calling the men in Traders ward, that's us, who wanted a request played for us. Unfortunately I was the only one who heard it in the ward as no one was in bed listening, as being 9.30 they were in the television room.

If it is fine tomorrow I will most likely call upstairs and thank Theresa for her request, though what it was I've no idea as I missed the actual tune, so will have to bluff it out. Apparently, St Helier Hospital Radio control this link, and one must phone them first in order to get any request played back to our end. I told Barry about the request, and he apparently knew the girl called Theresa and said he would see her in the morning. He noticed that Christopher was on the phone, and asked me to tell him when he had finished. I said I would wheel it along to his room. Christopher was certainly making lots of phone calls, which I learned later were to flog theatre tickets to his "customers", and it must have cost him a few pounds in change. I managed to signal to him that Barry wanted to use the phone, and learnt he had only one more call to make.

Had a glorious soak in the bath by 10.00pm and felt really refreshed after a rather sweaty day. Weighed myself again and found I was 55.4 kilograms, which was nearly 1 kilo lighter than before. I had hoped I would put on some weight, especially as I am eating so well.

Got to bed by 10.15 and had a sleeping pill for a change, to get off quicker. Lights went out at 10.30 - Goodnight all.

11. Friday May 14th

Roused at 5.30am. Good morning campers. Had a comfortable night thanks to the sleeping pill, though I did make a note of a visit to the loo at 3.45. It's the day for my stitches to be removed, so I'll be fussed over for a while later on, I hope.

Its just gone 6.00 and started to get socks and slippers on when I heard the rattle of the tea trolley. Nipped smartly to the top of the ward where Norma had already started pouring. Blotted my copy book somewhat with Norma when I mentioned that I was going to start at the other end for a change this morning. "You'll mess the system up" she said. "Start here and gradually work down as we get the temperatures and blood pressure done". I shrank back into my shell with slightly deflated ego.

Anyway, my practice yesterday served me well, as things went smoothly this time and I managed to get through the whole pot complete with second helpings by just topping up with hot water now and again. Finished exactly at 7.00. Made my menu out for Saturday and went through all 3 meals laboriously, then it suddenly dawned on me, I will only be here for the breakfast section, so had another try on a new form.

Just had a word from Bob that I dozed off last night, while writing up my notes for the day, sitting up with pen poised and eyes shut. Norma, the night nurse, put my light out and left me. Bob went on to say that half an hour later, I took my glasses off, put my writing things away and laid down. I remember doing all that but don't recall putting my light out, which all figures now. Did the sleeping pill have this effect on me.

Breakfast arrived at 8.00am with usual choice of cornflakes or porridge. I had both for a change in the hopes of putting back the 1kg I lost during the previous 36 hours, and followed by a boiled egg, bread and butter, as rolls were off today.

Saw some of the nurses again who had been away the last few days. They were pleased to see me so well. I started on my diary, when Bob opposite (still in bed) said "Hey Les, what are you doing?" I answered, "writing up my notes." "You're not supposed to be here, but in the day room with the other able bodied patients, because being Friday, it's floor cleaning day." No one had told me about this rule, then I recalled that last Friday when I was a bed patient, the cleaning gang came round and the beds were pushed to the centre of the ward, while the scrubber and polisher slid silently across the floor from side to side.

So here I am continuing my notes among the rest of the able bodied men reading their papers, while the monotonous drone from the extractor fan in the window above the TV set continues its whirring actions. This is the only sound being made in this room, broken occasionally by a rustle of someones newspaper.

It is now 8.40 and one or two registrars and other staff have been using the day room as a short cut to the ward in preparation for the doctors rounds at 9.30.

Began to feel the call of nature and anxious to return to the ward toilet. This was accomplished eventually and my bowel operation was perfect, no trouble there. Sat at my bed waiting for temperature, pulse and blood pressure to be taken, when staff nurse announced it's coffee time. Gladys retorted, "I haven't made it yet".

Managed to get a picture of Bob in his wheelchair holding a large yellow ribbon bow borrowed from someone's flower arrangement.

Final preparations were being made to bed

65

patients, and screens opened one by one in readiness far doctors rounds, which seem to have been delayed by the floor cleaning programme.

A sudden release of tension indicated that the expected doctors round had been cancelled for some reason. Hooray!

The nurse who is taking my stitches out came and informed me of the fact, and added, this is my first time at it. Hope she's gentle with me.

Gladys has just entered with coffee and teas trolley and while consuming mine, temperature, pulse and blood pressure were recorded.

My final thought for the day being another anagram of NIL BY MOUTH, turned out as "U BI MONTHLY" and this was displayed above my bed.

Have just been told my stitches are to be removed and to lay on the bed, and await developments. I must have been laying relaxed for half an hour before any action commenced, the time being 10.45.

I had been listening to a Robby Vincent phone in programme which had been very funny. In fact half way through the preparations, the head phones had to be removed in case any chuckle of mirth caused my tummy to bounce about, while Sue was in the act of removing the stitches.

The final stitch removed, all very painless, and after cleaning and disposing of dressings and other debris, checked time at 11.00. Well done Sue, assisted by Linda.

After a lovely soak in the bath, it was time for lunch, and the able bodied assembled to be served with our menus. I had beef curry and chips, lemon sponge and custard.

Another glorious day outside with a slight cooling breeze, so I hope to take some outdoor photos of some of the lads and any nurses, I can rope in. Took a photo of the ornamental pond while no one was around.

Latest thing now, is that I've got Bob hooked on this anagram lark and has come up with a good one for tomorrow.

Had a session outside with my tapestry until 2.15, then decided to come in and wait for Joyce, who arrived about 2.20. While waiting for Joyce, Tommy's mother, father and a sister came to take him home. He is the young lad who had an 'op' on his toe. I heard that there were 5 children in their family.

I was so pleased that Joyce agreed to come outside, as I did so wish her to meet the friends I've made here. It was so gorgeous in the shelter of the building with the sun feeling so warm and inviting. Bob and Dennis, their wives and friends were all out there and I was proud to introduce Joyce to them. We were all enjoying a good old natter, as though we had known each other for years. To make things even more perfect, the tea trolley came round at 3.00 and after Gladys had supplied the patients with their tea and biscuits, she managed to supply tea for our friends and Joyce, which was a lovely thought for the afternoon.

All too soon, however, the bell was rung, and there was no way we could pretend we hadn't heard it, because it was brought out to us and rung again.

Seeing Joyce to the passage, this time with a much lighter, happier heart, and saying my farewells to many of the visiting friends of other patients I had spoken with.

Went back into the sunshine and took a photo of Bob in "semi nude skin" and the big yellow bow across his tummy. Borrowed two nurses to join up with Barry, Andrew and Dennis for a group. Organised someone to take another group, with me in it this time.

While still outside continuing a nattering session, looked round when my name was called and there was brother in law Fred, and his wife Norma to see me. I was excited as a small child and was so pleased to tell them how well I felt. We chatted about the 'op' and I gave them a sneak view of my 'scar'.

I couldn't say enough to cover all my experiences in the short time they were allowed. I had to pass on my feelings to Norma and Fred when I told them they had made my day, and in fact everyone today had made it a day to remember. I saw them off to the passage, and on my way past my bed sister Sheila informed me, my tablets were to be taken. Showed Norma and Fred the "get well" cards I had received, then walked with them to the exit doors.

During Joyce's visit, she had thoughtfully brought in a large box of Quality Street as she realised I would not be able to get anything for the nurses till I got out. I had a brainwave before I gave the box to the ward sister, by putting a label across the lid reading NIL BY MOUTH. Hope they understood the gag.

Sheila, the ward sister, has just come back to thank me for the present to her and the nurses, and to wish me all the best for the future. She said she loved looking after me and to write any time, I feel in praising the nurses for their efforts, as it does boost their moral and encourage good results.

In no time at all, supper time appeared, but the serving was carried out by the ward sister and a nurse, because of a dispute which started yesterday affecting the normal ancillary staff. During the meal however, a deviation from the run of serving the food caused a hush over us, when we learned that the elderly gentleman in the first bed had just passed away. He had been there during the whole of my stay, and it was not all that long ago he had a few glum visitors sitting by his bedside. This put added strain on the sister, who appeared to take it all in her stride, on top of the extra work brought on by the dispute. When the meal was over we all mucked in and cleared the table, cleared up all the crocks and cutlery, and loaded the trolley ready for removal.

While resting on my bed, there was much activity going on around the deceased gents bed. The screens were round all the time and sister and nurses were popping in and out carrying out the necessary work.

Eventually a rumbling sound made me look up, and I observed a covered trolley appear, and guessed it was to take the gent on his 'ride' to the morgue.

Visiting time was approaching and all was cleared before they started through the ward, all of them passing the bed (still screened) where the old gentleman had been.

My tapestry must be finished tonight at the latest, and as there are only 7 rows to go, each getting shorter due to the curvature of the picture, it shouldn't be hard. Plugged away steadily and reached my goal just before the bell went.

Everything seemed quiet when the nurses brought the evening drinks round, and I thought everyone was watching TV. However, when I sauntered down to the day room and found the set off and no one there, I couldn't believe my luck. It was just after 9.00pm and I could see the "We'll Meet Again" serial without upsetting anyone else's programme.

Some of the lads trickled in during the evening and respected the fact that I was seeing the last episode. It certainly had been a lovely day for me, and after a quick wash, had a sleeping tablet and must have gone off quickly after the lights went out at 10.15pm.

12. Saturday May 15th

Awoke at 3.30am for a visit to the loo, and met Dennis on a similar errand. He's had lots of trouble with his piles, and has only just been cured.

Back to bed again and didn't re-awake until 6.00am and noticed Christopher opposite was already up and waiting by the tea trolley. I had delegated him as the "new" tea boy for the morning, and I'm sure he must have worried about it all night, because I've usually had to shake him awake.

When I realised I was no longer on the list for temperature and blood pressure, etc. I thought I might as well get up and assist Christopher who had already started the round. Between us we got through it double quick.

It's now 7.00am and I must have a wash and shave to be ready in good time for breakfast. By 7.30 all ablutions finished and wandered round the ward looking for an inspiration to use up my last films. Breakfast time came and went, the last one in this "holiday camp". Noticed the nurses already stripping my bed that had been my companion for so long. Started collecting my gear together and clearing out my locker, throwing out any old rubbish.

Just had a rousing "Happy Birthday" to Norman when it was discovered it's his birthday today.

Joyce and Chris, our next door neighbour at home, are due here at 10.00am with my going home clothes, so I am now waiting quietly for them to appear in the doorway.

Best news of the day was to be told by Bill in bed 1, that his tubes are out and he has "lost" his "pet bag". He certainly looks more perky now, and confessed to me that he cried a little with sheer joy when the final tube was removed.

A brainwave suddenly hit me in connection with Normans birthday. I confided to Bob about using a toilet roll with all our signatures on it, but when we tried a biro on the paper it wasn't successful. In any case on second thoughts it was a bit impersonal, especially when the nurses were required to sign it as well.

However, Bob came up with the idea to use a card that Charles had given him earlier. (Bob apparently collects old postcards and other cards). It seemed a suitable one with loads of flowers, and fortunately already had Charles' signature on it, especially as he was not in today. The job now was to gather as many of the men's signatures as possible and as many of the nurses as were on duty. When I first got chatting to Norman, a few days ago, he seemed to know me from somewhere and could not put his finger on where though. I told him I live at Banstead and he thinks he's seen me around the village.

The nurses had returned from their coffee break now and with frantic waving to attract their attention, the card was finally completed.

Countdown to my dressing time - 15 minutes, made a final wander round checking my bits and pieces were still intact on my chair, and stopping here and there with a word or two to the friends I'd made. Dressing time - 10 minutes.

Had a quick look up the passage to see any sign of Joyce, returned to the ward and had a word with Kathy my pet nurse, who asked me what I'd been writing about. Just couldn't resist letting her flip the pages over for the reactions to the snippets she read. She was enthusiastic and said she would like to read it all, no doubt to find out what I had said about herself. Many of the other nurses had mentions in parts, and I told Kathy you are the only one who has had a sneak preview, and if it ever becomes a paperback novel, it will be called "NIL BY MOUTH".

Dressing time - 5 minutes, and there was Joyce coming into the ward with my clothes. Nurses put screens round my bed and I started getting dressed, eager to be leaving at last. Heard voices saying Goodbyes and on looking out, saw Dennis all dressed up, who was also leaving today. Said my cheerio's to him and his wife, and disappeared behind the screens again for a final check. My dressing gown had to be carried in a separate bag that Joyce had thoughtfully provided, and with everything else packed in my case, I emerged like a butterfly from its cocoon and spread my arms in a wide arc.

Picking up my case and bags went to the end of the ward for a final handshake with Norman, who I notice had quite an array of cards around him. Continued along the row of beds shaking hands with many that still had some time to go before they to would be leaving, past the military gentleman Rudland or Les the "long one". I was Les the short one - a nickname by Bob, who else! Then the nurses had their farewell words of wisdom about not wanting to see me again unless I was only visiting.

Christopher promised to carry out his tea duties under new management together with Bill, who took over the number 1 bed when I was taken down the line to number 5.

Finally Kathy my sweet young blonde, who had my farewell kiss. A final look in the ward office for any lurkers, but it was empty. It was now 10.10 and Joyce had been patiently waiting while my next door neighbour Chris was in the car.

Out through the main doors, past the staff time clock - which momentarily reminded me of my work, and it was into the bright sunshine. It was so good to be alive and to enjoy such a beautiful setting as we walked to the car park. A parting farewell to Gladys, the tea lady and her helpers, and there was Chris ready by his car.

It was back to the wide open and sometimes cruel world I had previously left behind, while sheltering behind the protective care of the hospital and all its regulations, which I used to regard as petty and unnecessary before I came into the hospital system.

I know now from first hand experience how important is a proper kept timetable of regulations, the work involved in the running of an efficient hospital, and the dedication to their work of the Doctors, Surgeons, Sisters, nurses and ancillary staff who form such a large team. Thank you all.

THE END

ABOUT THE AUTHOR

Leslie J Curson, our late father, (1923-2004) was a Wireless Operator in the RAF during WWII.

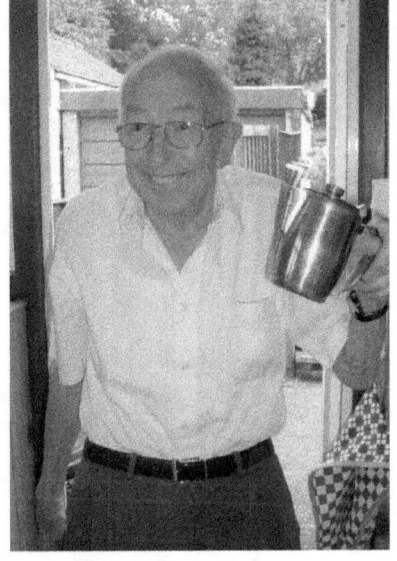

Apparently this is why he stood up when approached by Doctors in the book, you cannot take RAF rules out of a man after all those years.

After the war he worked as a Time Clock mechanic near London Bridge till his retirement at 65 years old in 1988. He was a warm and friendly man who always thought about helping others before himself.

Our father would have loved to know his book "Nil By Mouth" has now been published 13 years after his death.

David Curson - his son
Christine Paston - his daughter